Understanding
EPILEPSY

GW01003340

Dr Matthew Walker
Professor Simon Shorvon

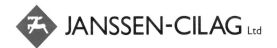

JANSSEN-CILAG Ltd

Sponsored by an unrestricted educational grant
from Janssen-Cilag Ltd

Published by Family Doctor Publications Limited
in association with the British Medical Association

IMPORTANT

This book is intended to supplement the advice given to you by your doctor. The authors and publisher have taken every care in its preparation. In particular, information about drugs and dosages has been thoroughly checked. However, before taking any medication you are strongly advised to read the product information sheet accompanying it. Your pharmacist will be able to help you with anything you do not understand.

© Family Doctor Publications 1995
Reprinted 1996

Medical Editor: Dr Tony Smith
Consultant Editor: Jane Sugarman
Cover Artist: Colette Blanchard
Medical Artist: Angela Christie
Design: Fox Editorial, Guildford, Surrey.
Printing: Reflex Litho, Thetford, Norfolk, using acid-free paper

ISBN: 1 898205 20 5

Contents

Introduction

What do the following people have in common: Julius Caesar, the apostle St Paul, Dostoievski, van Gogh, the prophet Mohammed, Joan of Arc, Buddha, Edward Lear, Gustav Flaubert and Alexander the Great? The answer is that they probably all had epilepsy. Similarly, today there are people from all walks of life who have epilepsy and it is therefore somewhat surprising that any misunderstandings arise. Indeed, fear of possible stigmatization or prejudice results in many people hiding their epilepsy from friends, employers and sometimes even family.

Epilepsy has achieved its unenviable position in people's minds, perhaps largely because of its unpredictable, dramatic and sometimes frightening effects. Although there are many different types of seizures, as will be explained later, it is the convulsion – the falling to the ground, the frothing at the mouth, the flailing of the limbs – that comes to most people's minds when the word epilepsy is mentioned. It is this dramatic event that has always fuelled people's imaginations; epileptic seizures are mentioned in the earliest Babylonian and Hebrew tracts. In Ancient Greece, at a time obsessed with gods and spirits, Hippocrates was one of the first to try to dispel the mysticism of epileptic seizures. He firmly believed that epilepsy originated in the brain and even went as far as condemning those charlatans who proposed that epilepsy was due to demonic possession.

Yet for the next 2,000 years, it was this theory of demonic possession that led to people with epilepsy being shunned, locked away and subjected to unpleasant, painful and humiliating ordeals in the name of a cure. In the account of the death of Charles II, there is a description of the treatment of his seizure; this included bleeding him, giving him substances that made him sick and repeated enemas, shaving his head, blistering his skin and then finally forcing an unpleasant concoction down the dying king's throat. Even as recently as the nineteenth century, circumcision and castration were proposed as cures of epilepsy. It was not until the end of the nineteenth century that the first effective drug, potassium bromide, was introduced, and from that time drug treatment has allowed the majority of people with epilepsy to lead normal, seizure-free lives. However, there is still, to a certain extent, a stigma attached to what is a common condition (almost every one of us knows someone who has epilepsy, although we may not know that he or she has the condition).

HOW WIDESPREAD IS EPILEPSY?

Epilepsy is very common. Each year in the United Kingdom about 25,000 people develop epilepsy, the majority being either children or elderly people (epilepsy infrequently starts between the ages of 20 and 50).

There is about a one in 30 chance of developing epilepsy during a lifetime. However, only one in 200 people has active epilepsy (300,000 people in the UK). This implies that most people with epilepsy get better, and indeed this is the case; in about six out of every ten people the condition resolves.

Epilepsy affects males and females almost equally, although certain types of epilepsy are more common in one or other sex. It affects all classes and all races. Thus epilepsy is common, and usually gets better; this is an important message for all those who develop the condition.

FACTS AND FIGURES ABOUT EPILEPSY

Out of 50,000,000 people (the approximate population of the UK):
    1,000,000–2,500,000 will develop epilepsy in their lifetime
    250,000–500,000 will have active epilepsy
    10,000–35,000 will develop epilepsy each year

KEY POINTS

√ There are many types of epilepsy and seizures

√ Epilepsy usually begins in childhood or old age

√ Epilepsy is common, but usually resolves

What are seizures and epilepsy?

Seizures (or fits; seizures is the preferred term, these days, and is thus used throughout this book) take many forms. They originate in the brain, and different types of seizures arise in different parts of the brain.

The brain is involved in forming emotions, thoughts, memories, in controlling movement and in appreciating sensations, sounds, smells, tastes and sight. The brain is divided into two halves joined in the middle; the right half controls the left-hand side of the body and the left half controls the right-hand side. For most of us, the left half is 'dominant', in other words, it controls how we form and understand language. Each half (or

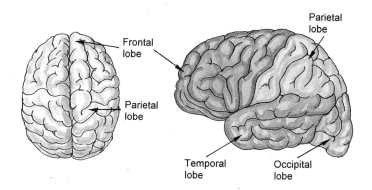

Anatomy of four lobes of the brain.

hemisphere) is further divided into four lobes as shown in the box.

LOBES OF THE BRAIN

Frontal – among other things, involved in the control of movement

Parietal – involved in the appreciation of sensation

Temporal – involved in the formation of memories and the appreciation of smells and tastes

Occipital – involved in vision

Damaging one part of the brain will take away its function. For example, damage to the left occipital lobe will result in the person being unable to see anything on the right; damage to the right frontal lobe will cause a person to be paralysed down the left-hand side. Conversely activating the left occipital lobe, for instance with electrical current, results in the person seeing coloured blobs on the right-hand side, and stimulating over the right frontal lobe causes the left part of the body to move.

A seizure can be likened to an electrical storm. This storm can be confined to one part of the brain, spread to other parts of the brain or involve the whole brain at once. Those that start in one part of the brain are known as 'partial seizures' and those that start in both halves at once are known as 'generalized seizures'. What a person experiences and what is seen by others depend upon where in the brain the seizure starts, and how far and how quickly it spreads.

In the next section we define the different types of seizure in some detail.

TYPES OF EPILEPTIC SEIZURES

Almost all seizures are sudden, short-lived and self-limiting. Most occur spontaneously without warning and, as explained above, the form of the seizure depends on the part of the brain involved. The classification is presented in the table.

CLASSIFICATION OF SEIZURES

I **Partial seizures**
  A Simple partial seizures
  B Complex partial seizures
  C Secondary generalized seizures

II **Generalized seizures**
  A Absence seizures (petit mal)
  B Myoclonic seizures
  C Clonic seizures
  D Tonic seizures
  E Tonic–clonic seizures (grand mal)
  F Atonic seizures

Partial seizures

• **Simple partial seizures:** these are seizures confined to one small part of the brain during which there is no loss of consciousness. They are often divided into temporal lobe, frontal lobe, parietal lobe and occipital lobe seizures depending on where the seizure starts.

In temporal lobe seizures, the patient may experience a feeling of intense fear, vivid memory flashbacks, intense déjà vu (a feeling of having been in an identical situation before) and unpleasant intense smells or tastes. We can all experience some of these from time to time and of course they are not usually seizures; for example, déjà vu is a common and normal experience. The main difference is that, with epilepsy, these things happen regularly, without reason, they are short lived and occur with an intensity that is rare in everyday life.

In frontal lobe seizures, there may be uncontrolled jerking of one arm or leg or the head and eyes may turn to one side.

In parietal lobe seizures, the patient may experience tingling down one side of the body.

In occipital lobe seizures, the patient may experience flashing lights in one half of the vision. The seizure usually lasts a matter of seconds.

• **Complex partial seizures:** these are really the next stage up from simple partial seizures, and the clue is in the word 'complex'. In these,

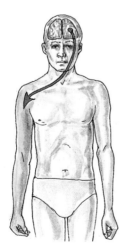

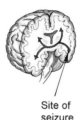

Site of seizure

Left partial lobe seizure affects right arm.

Temporal lobe seizure. It can spread causing generalized seizure.

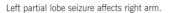

the seizure involves a larger part of the brain and spreads to enough of the brain so that the patient is no longer aware of his or her environment (i.e. becomes unconscious). The spread of the seizure can either be so fast that the patient does not experience the simple partial seizure or be slow enough for the patient to have, for example, a feeling of déjà vu, a strange unpleasant taste or an awareness of coloured flashing lights lasting seconds to a few minutes before becoming unaware of the surroundings.

During the seizure, it is common for complex, strange or inappropriate actions to occur (called 'automatisms'). For example, the patient may fumble with his clothes or make chewing movements. Occasionally, the actions are coordinated and can even take the form of running, dancing, undressing or speaking nonsense. These seizures usually last a matter of minutes, but are occasionally more prolonged. On coming round, the patient is completely unaware of what he or she has done.

• **Secondary generalized seizures:** these result from the spread of the seizure throughout both halves of the brain; the spread can be slow enough for the patient to have a warning (the aura, which is in fact a simple partial seizure) or so rapid that the patient loses consciousness without an aura. This spread is called secondary generalization and the seizure takes the form of a 'generalized tonic–clonic' seizure. In this, the patient often goes stiff (called the tonic phase) and will let out a high-pitched cry; he then falls, may go blue and his arms and legs jerk rhythmically (called the clonic phase), grunting can occur and he may foam at the mouth.

During the seizure the patient may bite his tongue or wet himself; it usually lasts a few minutes, and afterwards the patient is often confused, may not know where he is and will often sleep. The after-effects (the 'post-ictal' phase) last for minutes or hours. This seizure, which used to be called a 'grand mal' attack, is now known as a tonic–clonic seizure, and is also sometimes referred to as a convulsion.

Generalized seizures

These are seizures that begin in both halves of the brain at once; as such there is no warning and consciousness is lost immediately. Often this seizure is a tonic–clonic seizure (see above), but it can be a clonic seizure (no stiff phase) or a tonic seizure (no shaking stage, the patient just falls like a board). There is also a rare type in which the patient just slumps to the ground, but recovers quite quickly (an atonic seizure).

There are also two other categories of generalized seizures: absences and myoclonic jerks.

- **Absences:** these used to be called a 'petit mal' attack. They are short blank spells, usually in children, that last just a matter of seconds and can be confused with poor attention or loss of concentration. Children with absence epilepsy can have hundreds of these in a day and often neither the child nor observers are aware of most of them because they are so brief. They are associated with a particular brain wave pattern that is discussed in the next chapter.
- **Myoclonic seizures:** these are usually seen in patients with other seizure types, and are very brief jerks of one limb or the whole body. The patient may describe suddenly dropping a cup of tea as his hand flings up, or his whole body being thrown to the ground.

From this, it can be seen that there are many different types of seizure and already you are probably aware that there are other conditions that can be mistaken for a seizure and these will be discussed in the next chapter.

WHAT CAUSES SEIZURES?

All brain activity depends on the passage of electrical signals. The brain consists of millions of cells called neurons which have bodies and long arms with branches known as axons. It is down these axons that the electrical signals pass, like a telephone signal down a telephone line. When the signal reaches the end of the axon, it causes the release of a chemical; this chemical communicates with a nearby neuron body via special 'receivers' called

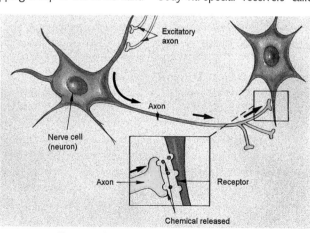

Diagrammatic representation of neuron and axon.

receptors. It may 'excite' this neuron body and if this excitation is sufficient then a further signal is sent (or 'fired') down its axon. This is the way in which the neurons communicate with each other. If only excitation took place in the brain, then eventually all the neurons would be firing together, so causing an 'electrical storm' such as seen in a seizure. But some neurons release a chemical from their axons that inhibits the surrounding neurons, stopping them from 'firing'. The brain functions properly when there is a balance between the excitation and the inhibition. If there is either too much excitation or too little inhibition in a part of the brain (an imbalance), a seizure results.

In partial seizures, the local imbalance between excitation and inhibition can be caused by local damage to the brain, for instance, from lack of oxygen at birth, meningitis or head injuries, or by abnormal tissue such as a brain tumour or a defect in brain development. In some cases, the reasons for the partial seizures are not always known.

In generalized seizures, the chemical imbalance affects a wide area of brain, and the brain often shows no obviously abnormal structures. This can be caused by drugs, alterations of the body chemistry, excessive alcohol, inherited or unknown factors. Thus epileptic seizures are a symptom of an underlying brain disturbance in the same way that stomach ache is a symptom of an underlying gut disturbance (e.g. food poisoning, ulcers, appendicitis, etc.).

WHAT IS EPILEPSY?

Epilepsy is defined as *a condition in which the person is prone to recurrent epileptic seizures*, so diagnosis is a measure of the probability of having epileptic seizures. If you have one seizure brought on by excessive alcohol, and then you become teetotal, the chances of having another seizure are very small and you would not be diagnosed as having epilepsy. If, on the other hand, you had a number of seizures because of a damaged part of your brain, the chances of having another seizure are very high; you would be diagnosed as having epilepsy.

The decision about whether a patient does or does not have epilepsy is not always clear cut. We all have a lifetime chance of having a seizure of about one in 30 (29 to 1 against for those who bet, i.e. 'an outside chance'), and we can considerably increase our chances of having a seizure by drinking excessively or taking certain drugs. Most doctors only diagnose patients as having epilepsy if they have two seizures within a year, because, in this instance, the chances of having a third seizure are probably over 80% (4 to 1 on, i.e. 'a sure thing').

The difficulty arises in patients who have had one seizure, and in this instance the doctor usually assesses the chances of another seizure aided and abetted by various investigations, and knowledge of the type of seizure and the cause. Most doctors in the United Kingdom would not usually treat one seizure, in contrast to doctors in some other countries (this just reflects the odds at which doctors in different countries start treatment).

The second difficult question is, if a patient is diagnosed as having epilepsy, how many seizure-free years must pass before he is no longer thought to have epilepsy? Unfortunately, there is no simple answer to this question, but it is certainly true that most people with epilepsy eventually stop having

FEATURES OF EPILEPTIC SYNDROMES

Epileptic syndrome	Features
Benign childhood epilepsy with distinctive EEG changes	Occurs between 2 and 14 years
	Can be inherited.
	Seizures involve face, throat and tongue, and consciousness is preserved
	Occasionally tonic–clonic seizures occur during sleep
	Typical EEG pattern
	Most get completely better and drug treatment is not usually necessary
Primary generalized epilepsy	Usually occurs in childhood or adolescence
	Can be divided into many different syndromes
	Can be inherited
	Seizure types consist of a combination of absences, tonic–clonic seizures and myoclonic seizures
	Seizures usually occur on or within a couple of hours of waking
	Typical EEG pattern
	Usually well controlled with valproate

seizures and thus should not be registered as having epilepsy (if someone has not had a headache for 10 years, it would be perverse to call him a headache sufferer).

It is important to bear in mind that epilepsy is a symptom and not a disease as such. A symptom is something experienced by patients, indicative of an underlying disease. This is the case with epilepsy, which should be considered as an indicator of some underlying brain problem. A wide spectrum of brain conditions can result in epilepsy.

What is an epilepsy syndrome?

A syndrome is a medical term referring to a specific condition in which characteristic groups of symptoms occur together. They are often named after the person who first described them. For example, West's syndrome consists of infantile spasms (the baby suddenly bends over) with a particular brain wave pattern and often mental handicap in babies aged between three and 12 months. Most go on to have difficult to treat epilepsy and mental handicap. This explains what occurs and what happens, but does not tell us the underlying cause of the seizures (there are, in fact, a multitude of causes of West's syndrome).

The most common epilepsy syndromes are benign childhood epilepsy with distinctive changes on the EEG and primary generalized or generalized epilepsies shown in the table.

KEY POINTS

√ Seizures in different parts of the of the brain produce different effects

√ Seizures take many forms and can be likened to electrical storms in the brain

Diagnosis of epilepsy

When a doctor first sees somebody with possible epilepsy, there are two questions that are addressed:

1. Does the patient definitely have epileptic seizures?
2. What is the cause of the epilepsy?

ARE THE SEIZURES EPILEPTIC?

Many conditions can be confused with epileptic seizures. In adults, the most common are syncope (fainting), migraine, hyperventilation and panic attacks and 'pseudo-seizures'. In children, other conditions that can also commonly be confused with epilepsy include breath-holding attacks and night terrors.

Syncope

Syncope is the medical term for fainting, and occurs when not enough blood gets to the brain. The most common mechanism of syncope is the classic swoon (the 'vasovagal' attack), in response to, for instance, seeing something unpleasant, experiencing excruciating pain or standing for a long period of time in a hot enclosed space. Occasionally syncope is due to a heart disturbance (for example, if the heart goes into an abnormal rhythm) or it can be precipitated by particular events (including coughing or urinating).

The classic faint is well known to all of us; the person feels dizzy, hot and sick, becomes very pale (a deathly white), his or her vision goes grey and then he or she slumps to the ground. At this point, the blood flow to the brain increases and the person comes round quite quickly. At first sight, it would seem difficult to confuse this with the seizures mentioned in the previous chapter. However, some jerking of the limbs can occur, especially if the person is propped up because this may stop enough blood reaching the brain. The jerking is occasionally prolonged, but seldom has the coordinated pattern of a tonic–clonic seizure. In some partial seizures, the person may experience similar feelings to those of a faint so that the two conditions are not always easy to distinguish.

Migraine

As most people are aware, migraines often begin with a disturbance in vision or can be associated with tingling in the arm or face, and rarely with a disturbance of speech. It can be difficult to distinguish this from a simple partial seizure, especially because it is not uncommon to have a splitting headache after a seizure. Consciousness is, however, practically never lost with a migraine. There are also differences in the disturbance of vision between that in migraine and that in epilepsy. In addition, if tingling is experienced, it tends to spread slowly up the arm in migraine and rapidly in seizures. In most cases, there is little doubt about whether an attack is caused by migraine or epilepsy, but occasionally it can present a diagnostic puzzle.

Hyperventilation and panic attacks

Overbreathing (hyperventilation) is not uncommon, especially in those under a lot of stress or in those who tend to panic ('panic attacks'). The immediate feeling is usually described as a sudden difficulty in catching one's breath, and a feeling of panic (although these do not always have to be present). During overbreathing, a person breathes out too much carbon dioxide and when this happens the acidity of the blood changes. This affects nerve activity and can cause tingling sensations, spasms of the hand, light headedness and even black-outs. These attacks are best treated with relaxation and breathing exercises.

Rebreathing into a bag during an attack enables a person to rebreathe the carbon dioxide that he is breathing out and so prevent or reverse the unpleasant effects of hyperventilation.

'Pseudoseizures'

These are often the most difficult to distinguish from true epileptic seizures. These attacks are 'all in the mind', although usually involuntary and occurring without any conscious motivation. Occasionally these attacks are 'put on', but for the most part the patient has little control and they can be likened to an emotional outburst. The patient may fall, appear to lose consciousness and then thrash around or lie motionless. These attacks often have some deep-rooted emotional basis, and may require psychiatric treatment. They do not respond to drugs for epilepsy. When it is difficult to tell these from an epileptic seizure, patients are admitted to hospital for close observation.

Breath-holding attacks

Unfortunately toddlers can hold their breath until they turn blue, and may resort to this if they do not get their own way. Usually the attack stops there, but occasionally a strong-willed toddler can hold his breath until he passes out. These do not require drug treatment, and the attacks usually stop of their own accord.

Night terrors

These affect children usually under the age of five years. A few hours after falling asleep, the child appears to wake, is terrified and cannot be comforted. In the morning the child usually has no memory of the night's events.

Although worrying, these are completely innocent and do not require treatment.

INVESTIGATIONS

The most important diagnostic tool is the 'medical history', the question and answer session that occurs between patient and doctor in the consulting room or surgery. The doctor will try to determine whether the episodes are seizures by asking for a detailed description of what happens, and obviously, as consciousness may be impaired, it is important that there is someone present who has seen an episode in order to help with the description (or even better a video of the episode).

The doctor will be interested in what the underlying cause of the seizures is and will thus ask questions about head injuries, problems with birth, whether the patient has had meningitis, alcohol consumption and whether other people in the family have epilepsy. He will also be interested in the impact that epilepsy will have on the patient's life and so will ask about the patient's job and home life. Lastly he will examine the patient looking for clues as to whether there is some underlying brain abnormality, and may also

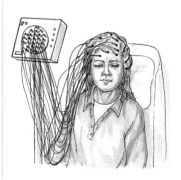

A patient has been prepared for EEG measurement.

check the heart especially if syncope is suspected.

A detailed neurological examination involves checking the eyes, the face, coordination, power and sensation in the limbs, and the reflexes in the arms, legs and feet. Besides blood and other routine tests, there are three special investigations that the doctor may decide to request which we will describe in some detail: electroencephalography (EEG), computed tomography (CT) scanning and magnetic resonance imaging (MRI).

EEG (electroencephalography)

This is literally 'recording the electricity from the brain'. Wires are attached to different parts of the head which are then connected to an amplifier; this amplifier magnifies the small electrical signal from the brain and records this signal onto paper. EEG is merely a recording of the internal electrical patterns of the brain, and as such does not involve

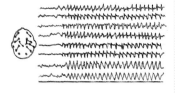

EEG showing recordings from different positions on the scalp during a burst of 3 per second spike/wave discharges associated with absence epilepsy.

the passage of any electricity into or out of the brain. It is thus a harmless and painless investigation, and is of great use to the doctor.

Normally, the tracing shows a wave pattern (the 'brain waves') with one wave occurring every tenth of a second or so. The waves slow down during sleep, and speed up when the patient is alert. If the patient is prone to epilepsy, the electrical pattern may be different, in particular showing what are called spikes or spike/wave patterns. Spikes can be picked up by an EEG performed in between seizures in about half the patients with epilepsy, but, if spikes are present, there is a 99% chance of the person having epilepsy. EEGs are occasionally performed during sleep because spikes are more likely to be picked up during this period.

A particular EEG pattern called a *3 per second spike and wave* is of particular importance. This is seen in patients with absence epilepsy, which has a specific form of drug treatment and a good outcome.

EEGs performed during a seizure, and especially if the patient is videoed at the same time, are of great use in patients in whom the diagnosis is in some doubt and in identifying exactly where the seizure starts (necessary, for instance, in assessing patients for epilepsy surgery). One such test is called video telemetry. This involves patients being admitted to hospital for several days during which they are constantly monitored by EEG and video. Sometimes it is also necessary to reduce or withdraw the patient's antiepileptic drugs to induce a seizure while the patient is being monitored.

CT scan

Computed tomography is literally the use of a computer to give pictures of 'slices' of the brain. This technique uses X-rays; however, unlike a conventional skull X-ray in which X-rays are fired at one side of the head, with a photographic plate on the other side, in a CT scan X-rays are fired at different angles and picked up by 'receivers'. The information obtained is then analysed by a computer which displays the X-ray signal as a series of pictures of slices through the skull and brain, something like slices through a loaf of bread. Using this technique it is possible to demonstrate such brain abnormalities as tumours, strokes or brain haemorrhages. However, CT is gradually being replaced by MRI (see below) in the diagnosis of the causes of epilepsy, because MRI is a much more sensitive test and gives much clearer pictures. During a CT scan the patient has to lie with his head stationary in the scanner for a number of minutes. This is an entirely painless procedure.

Occasionally a dye is injected into a vein in the arm to highlight certain parts of the brain in order to gain more information from the scan.

Magnetic resonance imaging (MRI)

This does not use X-rays at all. A large, powerful magnet is placed around the patient's head. The atoms in the brain orient themselves along this magnetic field. A burst of radio waves is then 'fired' at the patient and the hydrogen atoms in the brain wobble (resonate). As the hydrogen atoms gradually return to rest, they give off radio waves that are picked up by 'receivers' and analysed by a computer; this gives detailed pictures of the brain. This technique is very safe and entirely painless; however, it does involve lying in the scanner, which is an enclosed space, for some time (usually 10 to 20 minutes) which some people find unpleasant. Also, because powerful magnets are used, people with some types of metal implants (for instance, clips or wires from previous brain or other operations and pacemakers) cannot be scanned.

This technique can detect many subtle and small abnormalities that were previously undetectable by CT scanning. As MRI techniques improve so the underlying cause of epilepsy is being discovered in

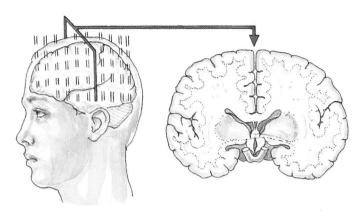
Brain scan.

more and more patients. MRI is especially useful in assessing the suitability of patients who have not responded to drugs for surgical treatment (see page 30). Also, using computer analysis, the relative size of different brain structures can be calculated. This is important in, for instance, analysing certain areas of the brain (especially an area known as the hippocampus) which, when damaged, can cause seizures.

CAUSES OF EPILEPSY

As has been emphasized, epilepsy is a symptom and not a disease. There are many causes such as infections, head injuries, brain tumours, brain injuries at birth and inherited diseases (see the table). Occasionally epilepsy can present many years after the damage has occurred. For example, it is not uncommon for people who have sustained a brain injury in childhood to present with epilepsy in their twenties. For many sufferers (about 70 per cent) no known cause is ever found. In the generalized epilepsies, genetic factors are likely play a role, and some epilepsies are hereditary, but in most cases this is not so (how do you inherit a head injury?). Except in a few genetically inherited conditions that can cause epilepsy, the risks of passing the epilepsy on to offspring are very small.

CAUSES OF EPILEPSY FROM BIRTH TO OLD AGE

Inherited brain diseases, e.g. tuberous sclerosis

Inherited epilepsies, e.g. primary generalized epilepsy

Birth trauma

Febrile convulsions

Brain infections, e.g. meningitis, encephalitis, brain abscesses

Recreational drugs and alcohol, e.g. cocaine, amphetamines, 'Ecstasy'

Head trauma

Blood chemical abnormalities, e.g. low calcium, magnesium or glucose

Cerebral haemorrhages

Brain tumours, e.g. gliomas, meningiomas

Strokes

Dementia, e.g. Alzheimer's disease

KEY POINTS

√ Many conditions are confused with epilepsy, the most common being fainting, migraine, panic attacks, 'pseudoseizures', breath-holding attacks and night terrors (the last two in children)

√ Epilepsy can be caused by infections, head injuries, brain tumours, brain injuries at birth, inherited diseases, but often the cause is not known

√ Investigations for diagnosing epilepsy include EEG, CT scan and MRI, but the 'history' is of greatest importance in making the diagnosis

√ Risks of passing epilepsy on to offspring are very small

Treatment of epilepsy

ON THE SPOT MANAGEMENT OF A CONVULSION

Seizures and convulsions are often frightening to watch, especially because the person may turn blue, have wild, jerking movements, foam at the mouth and cry out. People often wish to intervene by placing an object in the person's mouth to 'prevent him swallowing his tongue' and by calling an ambulance. The former intervention can, however, be dangerous; objects should not be placed in the patient's mouth during the convulsion, because the patient may bite the hand of the helper and bite the object resulting in damage to the teeth and mouth.

If you are subject to many seizures, having an ambulance called every time is embarrassing and usually unnecessary.

During a convulsion the patient should be laid on the ground away from objects that can cause injury, the head should be cushioned and the patient should not be restrained in any way.

After the convulsion, the patient should be turned on to his left side and someone should remain with the patient until he is fully recovered. Sometimes, confusion can mimic aggression. In these cases the patient should not be restrained, but gently coaxed out of danger. At this stage, if anything is blocking the airway, it should be cleared. If the convulsion lasts longer than ten minutes, or if the patient is having repeated convulsions without consciousness being regained, then an ambulance should be called.

Some patients have recurrent prolonged seizures, and occasionally carers will be asked to give these patients a drug called diazepam either by mouth or as a suppository in order to stop the seizure. This policy should be

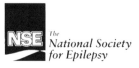

discussed with the doctor in charge of the care of any patient who has repeated episodes of seizures lasting longer than 20 to 30 minutes, because immediate drug therapy may be beneficial to the patient and prevent the patient needing to go to hospital.

LONG-TERM TREATMENT

The aim of long-term treatment is to stop all seizures, and this can be attained in most (about 80 per cent) patients. The following are the three main ways to achieve this:

1. Avoiding those things that cause seizures
2. Drug treatment
3. Brain surgery.

Very occasionally, patients who have warnings that last a long time before losing consciousness are able to control their seizure and prevent the loss of consciousness. This is sometimes achieved by intense concentration during the warning period.

Avoidance

In many patients, avoiding certain factors will lessen the frequency of seizures and in a few will prevent them altogether. Very rarely, people can have seizures brought on by hearing particular pieces of music, reading, hot showers, seeing certain patterns, etc. and these are referred to as 'reflex epilepsies'. For most, however, no specific trigger is ever noticed. There are nevertheless four things that can induce or worsen seizures in many: excessive alcohol, lack of sleep, stress and fever. Lastly, a few patients are sensitive to flashing lights (this is called photosensitivity (see page 21).

• **Alcohol and sleep deprivation:** often patients with primary generalized epilepsies are particularly susceptible to seizures following binges of alcohol or sleep deprivation, but these are almost certainly two factors that all people with epilepsy should try to avoid. Indeed, alcohol abuse or suddenly stopping a pattern of alcohol abuse can induce seizures in almost anyone, and seizures are thus a common complication of alcoholism. For those whose seizures are particularly exacerbated by sleep deprivation, getting tired, missing sleep and sometimes shift work are inadvisable.

• **Stress:** although it is often difficult to identify the effects of stress, it can nevertheless have a profound effect upon seizure control. Furthermore relaxation exercises, stress management and such therapy as aromatherapy can have a beneficial effect, and thus should be recommended to many patients. Often counselling those who have difficulties coping with their epilepsy can help seizure control. Depression, low mood and low moral can also increase the frequency of seizures. These factors can in addition affect how regularly patients take their medication (compliance), and thus indirectly worsen seizure control.

• **Fever and high temperatures:** during any illness seizures can get worse, and this is especially so in young children if a fever is present. This is because a high body temperature makes the brain more likely to have a seizure. Thus at the first signs of a fever, the body temperature should be kept down with regular paracetamol and, if necessary, a fan or cold sponging. Another instance in which the body temperature can increase resulting in increased seizure frequency is sunstroke, which is usually due to a combination of excessive sun exposure and dehydration.

• **Photosensitivity:** recently much has been made of light sensitivity (photosensitivity) and the relationship of seizures to video games, televisions or computer screen; in fact, less than five per cent of all people with epilepsy are sensitive to flashing lights. The photosensitive seizures usually occur with lights that flicker from five to 30 times per second and television and video games (both of which have flickering screens) can induce photosensitive seizures in susceptible individuals. However, children in the UK spend a large amount of time watching television and playing video games, and thus any seizure that occurs during this time may be purely coincidental.

Other common precipitants include:

• sunlight reflecting off water

- passing a line of trees through which the sun is shining
- stroboscopic lights (although local authorities do have guidelines on the flash rate of strobe lighting, it is perhaps best avoided by susceptible individuals).

In some patients with photosensitivity, avoidance of what triggers their seizures or taking certain precautions, such as the use of sunglasses in bright light, rather than antiepileptic drug treatment, may be all that they need to do to prevent the seizures. The following are the precautions that can be taken to avoid television-induced seizures for those not on drugs:

- viewing the television in a well-lit room
- viewing the television obliquely
- sitting at least 2.5 metres from the television set
- changing channels with a remote control rather than getting too close to the screen
- covering one eye and/or using high-frequency (100 Hz) televisions.

Seizures are rarely triggered by films seen in a cinema, and usually computer screens operate at a sufficiently high frequency to avoid provoking seizures. However, in both these instances, the content, if it consists of a changing geometric pattern at the correct frequency, can very occasionally provoke a seizure. Antiepileptic drug treatment is usually effective in preventing photosensitive seizures.

DRUG TREATMENT

Since the earliest times, people have been seeking effective drugs for epilepsy, and through the ages such cures as powdered human skull, vultures' blood and mistletoe have all been tried. The first effective therapy, however, was reported in 1857 by Sir Charles Locock, an obstetrician, who had an interest in epilepsy because of the mistaken idea, common at that time, that in some women epilepsy came from their wombs. The drug he used was potassium bromide, which was the most effective therapy until 1912 when pheno-barbitone was introduced. The main problems with bromides are their unacceptable side effects. In fact the play-off of side effects against the effectiveness of an antiepileptic drug is still at the heart of antiepileptic drug treatment.

What happens to a drug once it has been swallowed?

Once swallowed an antiepileptic drug is absorbed into the blood stream, passing into the brain which is where the drug acts. Whether an antiepileptic drug is taken on an empty or a full stomach can affect the amount of drug absorbed; they should generally be taken at the same time in relation to meals. Once the drug has passed around the blood stream it is removed from the body, either being broken down (metabolized) by the liver or filtered out by the kidneys and passed out in the urine (different drugs are removed in different ways). If a drug is removed from the body very quickly, then it has to be taken frequently (three to four times a day) to keep the blood levels reasonably high; conversely if a drug is only removed slowly then it can be taken once a day.

How do antiepileptic drugs work?

It is not certain exactly how most antiepileptic drugs work, but there do seem to be a number of important mechanisms. In an earlier chapter (see pages 8–9), it was explained that seizures may result when the excitation and inhibition occurring in the brain are not balanced. Some antiepileptic drugs correct this chemical imbalance. Other antiepileptic drugs work in a different fashion: they 'stabilize' neurons, and thus prevent excessive firing of axons.

Do all antiepileptic drugs work in all types of epilepsy?

Most antiepileptic drugs work in different types of epilepsy, and often it is just a matter of choosing the drug that suits the patient best. Interestingly, what may be a very effective drug in one patient may be useless in another. However, some antiepileptic drugs only work in particular forms of epilepsy (e.g. ethosuximide for absence epilepsy) and indeed some antiepileptic drugs can make some forms of epilepsy worse (e.g. carbamazepine for myoclonic seizures). A list of the drugs that are used most often in particular seizure types is presented in the table on the next page.

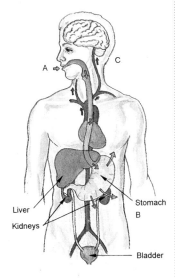

Stages of absorption: (A) drugs enter by mouth; (B) drugs pass from the stomach to the blood stream; (C) drugs pass to the brain in the blood stream. Then the liver breaks down some drugs and the kidneys filter some of them into the urine.

SEIZURE TYPES AND DRUGS USED

Seizure type	Drugs commonly tried first	Other drugs that are used
Partial seizures		
Simple partial	Carbamazepine	Acetazolamide
Complex partial	Phenytoin	Clobazam
Secondary generalized	Valproate	Gabapentin
		Lamotrigine
		Phenobarbitone
		Primidone
		Vigabatrin
Generalized seizures		
Absences	Ethosuximide	Acetazolamide
	Valproate	Clonazepam
		Lamotrigine
Atonic	Valproate	Acetazolamide
Tonic		Carbamazepine
		Clobazam
		Clonazepam
		Gabapentin
		Lamotrigine
		Phenobarbitone
		Primidone
		Phenytoin
Tonic–clonic	Carbamazepine	Acetazolamide
Clonic	Phenytoin	Lamotrigine
	Valproate	Phenobarbitone
		Primidone
Myoclonic	Clonazepam	Vigabatrin
	Valproate	Acetazolamide
		Phenobarbitone
		Primidone
		Piracetam

Side effects of antiepileptic drugs

There are three main types of side effects of antiepileptic drugs: dose-related, individual or idiosyncratic and chronic.

• **Dose-related side effects:** these are seen in all patients if the dose of the antiepileptic drug is high enough (this is sometimes called drug intoxication). The amount of drug that can be tolerated varies from patient to patient. With most of the antiepileptic drugs, dizziness, double vision, unsteadiness, drowsiness and headache are the most common dose-related side effects. They are alleviated by reducing the dose of the drug, but in the case of drugs that are removed slowly from the body, it may take several days for the effects of this to be felt. Importantly many people become used to some immediate side effects (especially drowsiness) after being on a drug for a little while, and thus it is always prudent to give a drug a month or so before abandoning it because of mild side effects. Most of the antiepileptic drugs can also interfere with concentration and intellectual ability.

• **Idiosyncratic side effects:** these are those that only occur in some people and are essentially allergies. They take the form of rashes or various blood disorders. As they do not depend on the dose of the drug, the only way to overcome these side effects is to discontinue the drug.

• **Chronic side effects:** these are the ones that occur after taking the drug for many years. The chronic side effects of the newer antiepileptic drugs are thus not as well documented as the chronic side effects of the older, more established drugs. The table includes the more common side effects that can occur with some antiepileptic drugs.

Drugs that interfere with antiepileptic drugs (drug interactions)

The blood levels of antiepileptic drugs can be affected by other drugs (including other antiepileptic drugs), resulting in either a fall in the blood level (causing seizures) or a rise in the blood level (causing side effects). This is because the

TYPES OF REACTIONS TO ANTIEPILEPTIC DRUGS

Idiosyncratic	Dose-related	Chronic
Rash	Double vision	Weight gain
Blood disorders	Unsteadiness	Vitamin deficiencies
Liver failure	Dizziness	Changes in facial
Psychosis/depression	Sleepiness	appearance
	Headache	Acne
	Stomach upset	Mood changes
	Slowness	Sedation

break down, excretion and absorption of antiepileptic drugs can be affected by other drugs. It is thus important to check before taking any other medication including those that can be bought without a prescription (see table for a list of some of the commonly prescribed drugs that interact with antiepileptic drugs). When a new antiepileptic drug is added to a patient's antiepileptic drug treatment, it is often necessary to change the dose of the existing antiepileptic drugs and to monitor blood levels.

Antiepileptic drugs can also affect the blood levels of other drugs. This is important for the contraceptive pill, because many antiepileptic drugs increase the body's ability to break down the pill, rendering it ineffective. In this instance higher doses of the pill are required. Breakthrough bleeding is a sign that the dose of the pill is probably not high enough, and that it will not be providing adequate contraception. A similar increase in drug metabolism occurs when antiepileptic drugs are combined with warfarin (a drug for preventing blood clotting), and this may result

COMMONLY PRESCRIBED DRUGS THAT INTERACT WITH ANTIEPILEPTIC DRUGS, AND THEIR USES

Drug	Use
Allopurinol	Gout
Aminophylline	Asthma
Amiodarone	Heart rhythm disturbances
Antacids	Indigestion
Aspirin	Pain killer
Cimetidine	Indigestion, peptic ulcers
Co-proxamol	Pain killer
Diltiazem	Angina
Erythromycin	Antibiotic
Fluoxetine	Antidepressant
Folic acid	Vitamin
Imipramine	Antidepressant
Omeprazole	Indigestion, peptic ulcers
Co-trimoxazole	Antibiotic
Verapamil	Hypertension

in the need for larger doses of warfarin.

Starting and stopping antiepileptic drugs

Starting antiepileptic drugs at a high dose can result in side effects. Thus antiepileptic drugs should be introduced cautiously and the dose increased in gradual steps. The final dose is determined by the balance between seizure control and side effects. It is important to realize that individual patients require different doses and that the final dose may be even more than the generally recommended maximum dose for the drug. In this instance, there is usually no need for concern if the patient is not experiencing side effects. If a drug does not work or if the side effects are unacceptable another drug is tried.

Most patients are controlled on only one antiepileptic drug (monotherapy – literally one therapy). In a smaller number of patients, two or more different antiepileptic drugs are necessary (this is called polytherapy – literally many therapies). For the following reasons the doctor will try, wherever possible, to avoid polytherapy:

- some antiepileptic drugs interact with other antiepileptic drugs
- side effects are often greater in polytherapy

- it is difficult to remember to take many different drugs and thus compliance is worse
- there is a greater potential for mistakes.

When a drug is being stopped, the dose must be decreased in gradual steps. A flurry of bad seizures can result from stopping an antiepileptic drug suddenly, even if the drug had not apparently been effective.

Compliance

Compliance is defined as the taking of a drug according to instructions received. Poor compliance (that is, failure to take a drug as instructed – either not taking the drug at all or taking it irregularly) is a major cause of the failure of antiepileptic drug treatment.

As it usually takes some time (days or weeks) for an antiepileptic drug to be fully effective, and seizure occurrence is usually unpredictable, it is imperative to take the drug regularly in order to prevent seizures. When patients are not having seizures they feel perfectly well (apart from the side effects of the antiepileptic drugs) and so it is thus not surprising that the occasional dose is missed either consciously or subconsciously.

It is also very easy for patients on regular medication to forget whether or not the last dose was

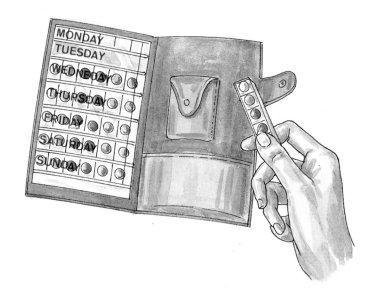

Drug wallet.

taken. It is important for patients to build up a regular routine of drug taking. Compliance is not helped if a drug has to be taken more than twice a day, especially in children who are not keen to take drugs midday at school. The situation becomes even worse if the patient is on polytherapy. A drug wallet with the tablets divided into different compartments according to the time of day and the day of the week is often very useful. All that then needs to be done is for the compartments in the wallet to be replenished each week. Drug wallets are also useful for those who have poor memories or very busy routines.

Occasionally patients decide to stop their drugs suddenly (often because of depression or low morale). This is potentially dangerous because it can lead to prolonged and frequent seizures. Also, during periods of vomiting or diarrhoea, the tablets may not be absorbed, and in these cases the tablets should be retaken or anti-sickness (antiemetic) drugs prescribed by the doctor; on occasion admission to hospital is necessary.

Last of all, misunderstandings between doctors and patients can lead to the wrong dosages being taken. After any consultation with the doctor it is important to be clear precisely how much of each drug needs to be taken; if necessary the doctor should write this information down. When coming for appointments, it is usually a good idea for the patient to bring the drug with him or her. Answers to vague enquiries about drugs are rarely helpful, for example, it would be impossible to give a response to 'Well, I take two blue or is it red pills in the morning, and then a white. No, I take the white pill in the evening'.

Monitoring antiepileptic drugs

It is important to monitor the effectiveness of an antiepileptic drug, and the best method is by seizure frequency. It is often surprisingly difficult to remember exactly how many seizures have occurred and thus a written record is mandatory for patients who have frequent seizures. This seizure diary can then be reviewed at each appointment with the doctor. It is important for patients to learn to differentiate between their different seizure types, and to record the frequency of each of them separately. Information of when antiepileptic drugs were started should also be included.

The most important guide to dosage is how well the seizures are controlled and how well or unwell a patient feels. However, occasionally it is helpful to take a blood sample (usually before the morning dose, although this is not always practical) in order to work out the blood levels of an antiepileptic drug. Much is made of blood levels, but it is important to keep these in context. The levels at which most patients

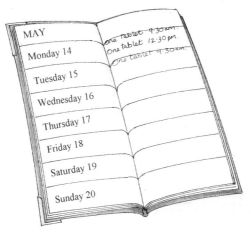

Diary page.

have good seizure control with few side effects give rise to the so-called 'therapeutic range' of blood levels for some antiepileptic drugs. The problem is that we are all individuals and what is an effective blood level for most people may be too high or too low for a minority. Blood levels can, however, give the doctor a rough idea of whether the dose of a drug is adequate.

There are also other circumstances in which blood levels are very useful:

- if poor seizure control occurs (blood levels may have fallen)
- to check for compliance
- if other drugs (including other antiepileptic drugs) that can interfere with the antiepileptic drug therapy are started
- during pregnancy and illness when drug levels may change
- in patients with severe learning difficulties who may not be able to communicate whether or not they are experiencing side effects.

The following chapter describes the various drugs available for treatment of epilepsy individually.

SURGERY FOR EPILEPSY

It has been estimated that about 12,500 patients with epilepsy in the UK could benefit from epilepsy surgery. The potential for and the success of surgery may increase as the technique called magnetic resonance imaging (MRI) improves and the cause of seizures can be identified in more and more patients. Epilepsy surgery is a major undertaking, because it involves removing the part of the brain where the seizures begin and obviously this is not without risk. Epilepsy surgery is therefore reserved for those patients with seizures resistant to drug treatment (also known as 'drug-resistant', 'refractory' or 'pharmaco-resistant' patients) and in whom there is little chance of the seizures improving.

Even before investigating patients for epilepsy surgery, several other criteria have to be fulfilled:

1. It has to be felt that the seizures are one of the main causes of a patient's disability (a severely handicapped patient may have uncontrolled seizures that are only a minor problem compared with the rest of his or her disability).
2. Similarly, it has to be felt by both the doctor and the patient that stopping the seizures would result in a significant improvement in the quality of life (undertaking brain surgery for instance in someone who is suicidal or severely depressed for reasons other than their

epilepsy or in whom the epilepsy is only of small consequence is obviously not to be recommended).

3. The patient must be able to understand the possible risks and benefits of the epilepsy surgery.

There are then several tests that have to be performed:

1. Brain imaging by MRI is used in order to identify brain abnormalities that may be the cause of the epilepsy. If no such abnormality can be detected, this does not preclude epilepsy surgery, but makes it considerably less likely to be successful and rarely worth pursuing.

2. Psychological testing is carried out in some detail. This involves a number of word tests, memory tests and drawing/constructing tests which elucidate the functioning of different parts of a person's brain. This is performed in order to identify whether any psychological problem or condition present is related to the part of the brain causing the seizures, the importance of this part of the brain for a patient's memory, speech, etc., and lastly as a baseline for comparison with psychology after the surgery.

3. Measurement of the brain waves by electroencephalography (EEG) also plays a pivotal role. Usually this involves a technique in which the brain waves are correlated with a video of the seizure in order to identify where the seizure starts. This is necessary to check that the abnormality seen on MRI correlates with the part of the brain producing the seizures.

4. A test called the sodium amytal test is also sometimes carried out. This involves injecting the anaesthetic agent, sodium amytal, into each side of the brain in turn; the injection is through a tube inserted into the main blood vessel in the groin and then passed up to the blood vessels supplying the brain. Although sounding quite unpleasant, it is a relatively painless and safe procedure. As a result of the injection each half of the brain is put to sleep in turn for a few minutes. During this period, the patient's memory and ability to name objects are tested. Failure to complete the tests accurately means that the half of the brain put to sleep controls language and memory. In most people language resides in the left half of the brain and memory in both, but in a few people this pattern is lost. This is important to know,

because the effects of brain surgery on speech, understanding and memory are vital factors in deciding whether surgery is indicated and what type of operation is possible.

5. Lastly it is common for a psychiatric assessment to be performed in order to confirm that there is no mental illness present which would prevent the patient from having brain surgery (e.g. very severe depression) and which needs to be treated before surgery is performed.

Once all this information is available, the patient's hospital doctors and the brain surgeon meet to discuss the risks and benefits of epilepsy surgery for each individual patient. Once this has been decided, the risks and the likely benefits are put to the patient who then has to make a decision.

Outcome of surgery

The outcome for epilepsy surgery depends largely upon the type of operation, the part of the brain involved and the underlying cause of the epilepsy.

In patients with an identifiable defect in the temporal lobe of the brain (the most common situation), about 70 per cent will become seizure free following surgery, and another 20 per cent will have some improvement. This does, however, still leave one in 10 who has no improvement or who may be worse. Nevertheless, with improved imaging and surgical techniques, the outcome of epilepsy surgery continues to improve.

KEY POINTS

√ Aim of long-term treatment of epilepsy is to stop seizures

√ An antiepileptic drug is chosen to suit the patient

√ Side effects of drugs can be dose-related, occur in only some individuals or occur only in the long term

√ Some patients with epilepsy benefit from brain surgery

Drugs used in treatment of epilepsy

ESTABLISHED DRUGS

Carbamazepine

This drug has been around since the 1950s, and has been found to be both safe and effective in partial epilepsy and tonic–clonic seizures. It can, however, worsen absences and myoclonic jerks. Occasionally a rash or abnormalities of blood counts can occur which may mean that the drug has to be stopped. Too high a dose can lead to double vision, nausea, headache and drowsiness. Carbamazepine is also available as a slow-release preparation (once swallowed, the drug is only slowly released from the tablet), which can be taken less frequently and has fewer side effects.

Clonazepam

This drug is one of a group of drugs called benzodiazepines (others will be mentioned later), which are better known for their use in anxiety and as sleeping tablets. This drug is effective in absence seizures and other forms of epilepsy. However, in some patients the drug ceases to be effective after a period of time (usually about three months); this phenomenon is called tolerance. Like all benzodiazepines drowsiness and behavioural changes (especially aggression in children) are the main side effects.

Ethosuximide

This drug is only useful in absence epilepsy. Some patients develop a rash, and side effects include stomach ache, tiredness, headache and dizziness.

Phenobarbitone

This is one of the oldest established antiepileptic drugs, having been used since 1912. It is cheap and effective in most types of epilepsy, but in recent years it has grown out

Drug (trade name)	Year of introduction
Phenobarbitone (Gardenal)	1912
Phenytoin (Epanutin)	1938
Primidone (Mysoline)	1952
Ethosuximide (Zarontin)	1960
Carbamazepine (Tegretol)	1963
Diazepam (Valium)	1973
Clonazepam (Rivotril)	1974
Valproate (Epilim)	1974
Clobazam (Frisium)	1982
Vigabatrin (Sabril)	1989
Slow-release carbamazepine (Tegretol Retard)	1989
Lamotrigine (Lamictal)	1991
Gabapentin (Neurontin)	1993
Slow-release valproate (Epilim Chrono)	1993
Topiramate (Topamax)	1995

of favour due to its side effects. Originally it was used as a sleeping pill; it is thus not surprising that some people become drowsy, although this drowsiness is slight and usually improves with time. Paradoxically, it can have the opposite effect in children, and make them hyperactive and aggressive. In a few, pheno-barbitone can cause a rash and blistering. Too high a dose leads to drowsiness, impotence, depression and poor memory. With long-term use, phenobarbitone can coarsen facial features and decrease the body's stores of certain vitamins (folic acid and vitamin D).

Phenytoin

This drug has been in common usage since 1938. It was initially seen as a breakthrough because it was as effective as phenobarbitone but caused less drowsiness. Phenytoin is effective in partial seizures and tonic–clonic seizures. Some patients get a rash, in which case it should be stopped. Too high a dose can lead to dizziness, increased seizures, drowsiness, unsteadiness and double vision.

Long-term use can lead to swelling of the gums, coarsening of facial features, acne, facial hair and a decrease in the body's stores of certain vitamins (folic acid and vitamin D). Because of these long-term side effects, young people are not keen to use phenytoin and often a different antiepileptic drug is preferred.

Primidone

This drug is broken down in the body to phenobarbitone, and thus has the same side effects and uses as phenobarbitone.

Valproate

This drug was discovered to be useful in epilepsy purely by chance in France in the 1960s. It is now the drug of choice for light-sensitive epilepsy, myoclonic seizures and absences. It is, however, effective in all types of epilepsy. It needs to be used cautiously in children under the age of three years, when it very occasionally causes severe liver damage. Some people can get a drop in the number of platelets in the blood (these are necessary for blood clotting).

The most common side effects, however, are stomach upset, hair loss, tremor, swelling of the ankles, weight gain and drowsiness (especially if given with pheno-barbitone). Valproate is available as a slow release preparation.

THE NEWER DRUGS

When antiepileptic drugs are first developed, they are tried on patients with uncontrolled epilepsy (usually partial epilepsy) as add-on therapy to existing antiepileptic drug courses. If they prove to be successful, then initially they are licensed just for this purpose. Some new antiepileptic drugs are, however, effective in types of epilepsy that fall outside the scope of the licence and doctors are permitted to prescribe drugs for such conditions, but usually discuss this with the patient first.

Gabapentin

At present, gabapentin is only licensed to be used in partial epilepsy in combination with other antiepileptic drugs. It has few side effects, but at higher doses can cause dizziness, tremor and drows-iness; the frequency of seizures can also increase in some patients. The drug can also result in weight gain.

Lamotrigine

This drug originally had the same restricted licence as gabapentin, but can now be used as monotherapy. It is potentially useful in most types of epilepsy. In a few patients, it causes a rash and this seems to be more likely to occur if a patient is started at too high a dose. Too high a dose causes drowsiness, double vision and dizziness.

Topiramate

This is the most recent antiepileptic drug to gain a licence in the UK as add-on treatment for use in partial epilepsy. Its side effects usually occur on starting treatment and include tiredness, stomach upset, unsteadiness and rarely kidney stones.

Vigabatrin

This drug is only licensed for partial epilepsy in combination with other antiepileptic drugs. However, it may also have some use in other forms of epilepsy in children. About one in 20 people get depression as a side effect of the drug, and occasionally confusion or psychotic symptoms can occur. Other side effects such as drowsiness and dizziness are usually mild. Some patients also put on weight while taking vigabatrin.

OTHER DRUGS

Acetazolamide

This drug is a diuretic (a drug that makes you pass more urine), and is mainly used to treat glaucoma (an eye condition). It is, however, occasionally used as additional medication for patients with epilepsy and, in some, it can be very effective.

The main problem is that after a few months tolerance develops (i.e. it loses its ability to work) in some

patients; it can also cause a rash. The other main side effects are excessive thirst, tingling in the hands and feet, tiredness and loss of appetite.

Clobazam

This is a benzodiazepine (see Clonazepam above). It may be very effective in most types of epilepsy as an additional medication, but again tolerance develops in some patients after a few months. It is occasionally given intermittently (that is, for three or four days at a time) in those whose seizures occur in small groups (clusters) or at set times (for example, at the time of menstruation), or on days when it is particularly important to avoid a seizure.

Diazepam

This drug is also a benzodiazepine and it is not usually used as regular medication, but as a one-off in order to stop a long seizure. For this purpose it can be given by mouth or by suppository by carers or family. In hospital, it can be given by intravenous infusion (i.e. directly into a vein) to stop prolonged seizures.

Vitamins and diets

There is little evidence that either of these help seizures. Vitamin supplements may, however, be necessary for those on long-term antiepileptic drug treatment, because some antiepileptic drugs (see above) can interfere with the body's vitamin stores. Supplementary folic acid is also recommended for those who wish to get pregnant.

There is a particular diet called a ketogenic diet which may help seizure control in some children with severe epilepsy and mental handicap. Unfortunately this diet is unpleasant and difficult to maintain, and so is rarely used.

DRUGS FOR THE FUTURE

There are at present many studies taking place throughout the world of potential antiepileptic drugs (at the time of writing, at least ten new compounds look quite promising). This is encouraging for the future of antiepileptic drug treatment. However, no drug so far has proved to be a cure-all, and one of the unanswered questions for epilepsy research is why only some patients respond to only some drugs. Nevertheless, each new drug enables a greater number of patients to have a significant improvement in their epilepsy; it is hoped that, with a greater armoury of drugs, fewer people will have uncontrolled seizures.

The newer drugs may have fewer side effects than the older drugs, but it is important to realize that long-term side effects of new drugs may be unrecognized in contrast to those of older drugs, some of which have been around for over 50 years.

Special situations

FEBRILE CONVULSIONS

This term is usually reserved for convulsions that occur in young children (three months to five years) only at the time of fever ('febrile'). Febrile convulsions are of importance because they are common and often frightening. It should not, however, be referred to as epilepsy, because the condition almost always resolves as the child grows older.

It is sometimes necessary to exclude brain infections such as meningitis as a cause and occasionally a 'lumbar puncture' (a needle is inserted into the spine of a child in order to withdraw some of the fluid that surrounds the brain) is needed to make sure that there is no brain infection. In most cases there is no meningitis or other serious cause.

Indeed, over three per cent of children between the ages of three months and five years will have at least one seizure associated with fever without underlying brain disease. It is more common in those with a relative who has had similar seizures or who has epilepsy. One-third of children who have a febrile convulsion have subsequent febrile convulsions, but a very small number (less than five per cent) go on to develop true epilepsy.

If a child has had a convulsion with fever, then in future febrile episodes the child's temperature should be kept down with paracetamol and cold sponging. In very susceptible children diazepam suppositories can be given at the time of a fever to prevent another convulsion, and very rarely a child may need regular antiepileptic medication, usually with valproate or phenobarbitone.

STATUS EPILEPTICUS

Most seizures only last a few minutes. Some, however, can go on for longer – sometimes hours or even days. This is referred to as status epilepticus, which is defined as a seizure or a series of seizures lasting more than 30 minutes in which the patient does not regain consciousness. This can apply to all seizure types; tonic–clonic status epilepticus (usually called convulsive status epilepticus) is of most importance because it is a medical emergency.

As many as ten per cent of patients with convulsive status epilepticus die (usually not as a result of the epilepsy itself, but of the serious underlying cause of the status epilepticus, e.g. meningitis, stroke or malignant brain tumours). About half the patients with status epilepticus have had chronic epilepsy; in these cases sudden withdrawal of the antiepileptic drug is one of the most common identifiable causes. About half the patients have convulsive status epilepticus as their first seizure. When it occurs urgent hospitalization and emergency, intravenous, antiepileptic drug therapy are required.

Many patients have increasing numbers of seizures throughout the day leading up to the convulsive status epilepticus, and in some (certainly those in whom status epilepticus occurs regularly) diazepam given by mouth or suppository will prevent the occurrence of the status epilepticus. Such a contingency plan needs to be made between the doctor and the carers or family of the patient.

The other, non-convulsive types of status epilepticus are not as serious. Often the patient will just have a prolonged typical seizure or series of seizures, leading to

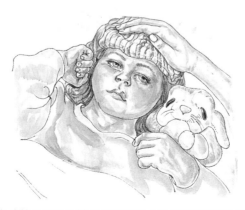

In children prone to febrile convulsions, keep the temperature down.

confusion which can go on for days. Non-convulsive status epilepticus usually responds well to medication given by mouth (often diazepam).

PREGNANCY AND EPILEPSY

Conception

Patients with epilepsy have lower birth rates. This is mainly due to social pressures, although epilepsy and its treatment can occasionally affect fertility. Furthermore, some antiepileptic drugs may decrease sexual drive.

The effectiveness of the contraceptive pill can be reduced by antiepileptic drugs and higher doses of the pill may be necessary in order to provide adequate contraception. Bleeding between menstrual periods is a useful sign that the oral contraceptive is not working.

Pregnancy

During pregnancy, about 30 per cent of patients experience an increase in seizures, 20 per cent experience a decrease in seizures and 50 per cent experience no change. The way the body deals with antiepileptic drugs is different during pregnancy, and regular monitoring of drug levels and seizures is often required. Quite often the dose of antiepileptic drugs has to be changed at some point during pregnancy. It is not uncommon for the mother to decide to reduce her medication during pregnancy because of a concern about the effects of the antiepileptic drugs on the developing child. Major, convulsive seizures can, however, damage the developing child or result in miscarriage, and thus the importance of good compliance cannot be over-emphasized.

The risks of antiepileptic drugs to the development of the baby in the womb are small. The risk is higher in infants born to mothers on polytherapy and on high doses of antiepileptic drugs. The overall frequency of abnormalities of the baby at birth is about two per cent for the general population, six per cent for babies born to mothers on one antiepileptic drug (i.e. still quite small), and up to 20 per cent for babies born to mothers on three different antiepileptic drugs (i.e. quite high). Thus, before getting pregnant, it is important for the doctor to get the patient on to the least amount of medication for adequate control of the epilepsy.

The most common significant abnormality in infants born to mothers with epilepsy is cleft lip/palate, which accounts for about one-third of the abnormalities seen. Spina bifida, the more serious side effect of drug treatment, is most common when the mother is taking valproate (1–2 per cent of births) or carbamazepine (0.5–1 per cent of births). Patients on these drugs can have ultrasound and blood tests during pregnancy to detect spina bifida early enough for the pregnancy to be safely terminated if the parents wish. All women on antiepileptic drugs should be given folic acid tablets (this is a naturally occurring vitamin) before conception and throughout the first three months of pregnancy, because this reduces the risk of miscarriage and fetal malformation, especially spina bifida (there is an argument for all women to take folic acid during these periods regardless of whether they have epilepsy or not).

In the last month of pregnancy vitamin K supplements should be given to the mother, and the newborn child should also receive vitamin K because antiepileptic drugs decrease the amount of this vitamin in the body. If the newborn child does not have enough vitamin K, then the blood may not clot properly, and there may be problems with bleeding and brain haemorrhage.

Breast feeding

Women with epilepsy on anti-epileptic drugs usually can safely breast feed, because with most antiepileptic drugs very little is passed out into breast milk. The exceptions are high doses of ethosuximide or phenobarbitone, which are excreted in breast milk in significant quantities; phenobarbitone excreted into breast milk can make the baby drowsy.

KEY POINTS

√ Convulsions that occur in young children only at the time of a fever do not usually lead to epilepsy

√ Seizures that last for hours or days are known as status epilepticus. and convulsive status epilepticus is a medical emergency

√ During pregnancy the risks of antiepileptic drugs to the baby are small, and certainly smaller than the risks of having uncontrolled convulsions

√ It is generally safe for women to breast feed while taking these drugs

Social implications

Although we have spent a large part of this book dealing with the medical aspects of epilepsy, it is important to realize that there are many social implications of epilepsy, for instance in regard to driving, schooling, employment and relationships. Unfortunately, society still places extra pressures on those who have epilepsy, sometimes with some justification as in the case of driving.

DRIVING

Seizures while driving are still one of the most common preventable causes of road traffic accidents. The rules laid down about driving are straightforward, and there is little excuse not to follow them. It is the obligation and responsibility of every person who has any condition that may impede his or her driving (this includes all people with epilepsy) to inform the Driver and Vehicle Licensing Authority (DVLA).

Anyone who fails to inform the DVLA, and continues to drive is committing a criminal offence. Furthermore failing to inform the DVLA may invalidate the driving insurance. This applies to all people with seizures, and for this purpose even the smallest epileptic event (for example, an aura or a myoclonic jerk) is counted as a seizure.

Once the DVLA has been informed, the patient should stop driving and can reapply for a licence only when one of the criteria in the box has been fulfilled.

- No epileptic attacks while awake (including aura, etc.) have occurred during the last year.
- If epileptic attacks have occurred, these were only during sleep, and this pattern has been present for at least three years.

Following a single epileptic seizure or if there is loss of consciousness of no known cause, patients can also be barred from driving for one year. When reapplying for a licence, it is necessary for the patient to fill in a detailed form about the attacks, and the DVLA can also seek information from the patient's GP and hospital specialist. If any person is unhappy with the DVLA's decision, it is possible to appeal through a Magistrates' court.

If a patient has been seizure free and has thus regained his driving licence, but wishes to come off medication, it is advised that the patient should not drive during the changes in medication and for six months after the withdrawal, although this is not legally binding. Unfortunately a seizure that occurs while coming off medication will result in loss of the licence.

The rules for heavy goods vehicle (HGV) and passenger carrying vehicle (PCV) licences are much stricter, and it is not possible to hold these licences if a person has a continuing liability to epileptic seizures. This is interpreted as meaning no epileptic seizure or antiepileptic medication for the previous ten years and no medical evidence of a continuing risk of seizures (e.g. three per second spike and wave on the EEG or a brain abnormality on brain scan).

EMPLOYMENT

There are a few occupations that are barred by statutory provision for people with epilepsy:

- aircraft pilot
- ambulance driver
- taxi driver
- train driver
- merchant seaman
- working in the armed services, fire brigade or police.

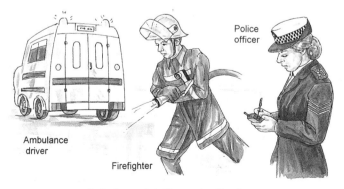

Police officer

Ambulance driver

Firefighter

Professions excluded for people with epilepsy.

There are also certain jobs that involve substantial risks if a seizure should occur and thus cannot be recommended (e.g. scaffolder), and commonsense should apply when considering such jobs. Furthermore there are jobs in which epilepsy is not explicitly mentioned but may be considered a bar (e.g. midwifery).

Patients are under an obligation to tell employers if they have epilepsy, if this could affect their ability to do the job or affect their safety at work. Failure to disclose epilepsy in such circumstances can be used as grounds for dismissal. If a seizure is likely to occur at work, it is, in our view, probably better to tell an employer rather than keep the epilepsy secret. If an employer is aware of a person's epilepsy and takes it into consideration then the work insurance will cover that person regardless of his condition. It is important to tell a workmate if a seizure is likely to occur at work, and to explain what to do if a seizure should occur.

When initially applying for a job, unless the epilepsy is likely to have a severe effect on the ability to do the job, there is no obligation to inform possible employers unless specifically asked. If asked on forms, it is important not to over-emphasize the epilepsy and in some cases it may be advisable to leave that section blank or to write that it will be discussed at interview.

The best moments for mentioning epilepsy are just before accepting the job offer or at final interview, but again it is important to try to place it in a favourable light. Often a letter from the GP or hospital doctor helps. The prejudice perceived by people with epilepsy when applying for jobs is probably often greater than the actual prejudice. Some people blame their failure to get work on their epilepsy when in fact the problem lies more in the person's attitude; it is essential at interview to appear confident, and appropriate for the job, rather than dwell too much on the negative aspects of epilepsy.

RISKS

One of the most important features of epilepsy is that it is an intermittent condition. If someone has a seizure once a week (this would be considered as poorly controlled epilepsy), it still leaves 313 days in a year when the person is seizure free. It is thus important that a person does not let the epilepsy take over and dictate his or her life. Overprotection, excessive restrictions and underachievement are far too common secondary handicaps of epilepsy, which can be avoided.

The main dangers from epilepsy come from its unpredictability, and certain precautions need to be taken.

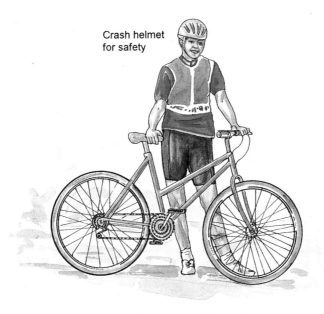

Risks for people with epilepsy – suitable attire for cycling.

It would be prudent to avoid certain high-risk situations such as mountain climbing, scuba diving and hang-gliding (although well-organized mountain climbs are possible). In most other circumstances the social and psychological damage done by restricting a person's life probably outstrip the risks. Swimming is perfectly possible, but preferably with someone who knows about the epilepsy and knows what to do should a seizure occur, and the pool attendant should be informed. Cycling and horse riding are perfectly possible, but again attention should be paid to the possible risks; both these pursuits need to be done either with someone who knows about the epilepsy or in an organized group, and a helmet is mandatory.

At home, most activities carry only a small risk. There are, however, certain actions that can be taken to minimize these risks. Showers should be preferred to baths and, if a bath is taken, it should be shallow and someone should be informed. Additionally, the bathroom door should remain unlocked. A microwave is preferable to a cooker, and pans of hot oil should be avoided. Guards for open fires, radiators and cookers

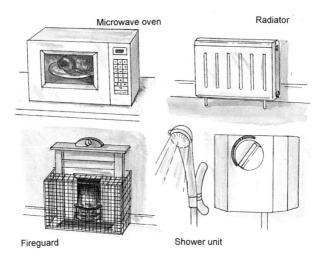

Microwave oven

Radiator

Fireguard

Shower unit

Household items for use by people with epilepsy.

are advisable. Lastly there are alarms that are available for people with epilepsy, which are triggered if, for example, the person falls; these are useful for people with frequent seizures who are living alone.

Frequent falls in someone with poorly controlled epilepsy can cause head and facial injuries. If these falls continue for long enough then a certain amount of brain damage and facial scarring can occur. In these people (very much the minority of people who have epilepsy), a protective helmet is advisable.

SCHOOLING AND PARENTING

It is wrong to generalize about a child with epilepsy. Epilepsy, as we hope is now apparent, describes many different conditions, has many different underlying causes and occurs in many different people. It is inexcusable to label a person with epilepsy as an epileptic child or an epileptic adult, and thus to suggest a stereotype. Despite this, there are some important points about schooling that need to be made.

Most children with epilepsy attend normal schools, and only the minority, who have epilepsy and learning difficulties or very severe epilepsy, need to attend special schools (advice about these is available from a number of organizations – see Useful Addresses on pages 54–5). Despite attending mainstream education many children with epilepsy underachieve at school for a variety of reasons. Epilepsy itself and antiepileptic drugs can impair a child's ability to learn. However, with modern drug management, there is less impairment of memory and greater control of seizures. A child with absence epilepsy can have many seizures that are unrecognized by both child and teacher, but which can present as lapses of concentration and poor class performance. Seizures at night can also affect performance during the day. More importantly, many children with epilepsy are almost expected by some to perform poorly, and this expectation by parents and teachers soon becomes self-fulfilling. Poor school attendance, low self-esteem and anxieties about school are all likely to be major factors. There has to be good communication between school, parents, child and doctor. It is important that the school knows about the epilepsy, that teachers know what to do about seizures and that they understand a child's condition. Education packages for schools are available from a number of charitable organizations (see Useful Addresses).

In addition, it is important that neither teachers nor parents restrict the activities of a child unnecessarily (see section on risks). The child should be encouraged to think positively and to take part in school activities. Teachers should be aware of possible teasing and bullying. If it is likely that a child will have a seizure at school, then often it is worth educating the class about seizures and epilepsy. It is important that the child does not feel or indeed become isolated because of his or her seizures.

Over-protection by families, even in well-controlled epilepsy let alone in poorly controlled epilepsy, is very common and is counter-productive. This over-protection, which often persists into adulthood, can result in social isolation, poor social graces, dependency, childishness, underachievement and low self-esteem. Striking a balance is understandably difficult, but it is important that this issue is not ignored. Parents should not be afraid to discuss their child's epilepsy with doctors, counsellors or others in order to have a better understanding not only of their child's epilepsy, but also of the restrictions that this will impose upon their child's life. In our experience, parents tend to verge much too much on the side of over-vigilance and over-anxiety, and thus the potential for psychological and social damage is great.

MARRIAGE AND RELATIONSHIPS

In broad terms, people with epilepsy have fewer relationships and are often more isolated than is normal. Prejudice among the general public is often blamed, but the actual causes of this are more complex. Some patients believe that there is a greater prejudice than actually exists. This in combination with parental over-protection can lead to a fear of relationships, and this anxiety often makes forming relationships more difficult. This results in a certain amount of social isolation which serves to fuel the original anxieties. We often find that these worries remain even when patients become seizure free. Many people with epilepsy thus need to be encouraged to think positively about themselves and their condition, and to face their anxieties. Occasionally help is needed, and advice about this is available from a number of sources (see Useful Addresses on pages 54–5). It is important not to let epilepsy dominate one's life inappropriately, as such a preoccupation can be very self-destructive.

Once in a relationship, if the epilepsy is still active it is important that the partner is aware of this. There is no evidence to suggest that knowledge of a person's epilepsy is a major cause in the break up of relationships. Although this may sound an obvious recommendation, we are certainly aware of one

person whose wife discovered about his epilepsy for the first time during a honeymoon night. How and when to tell a partner can be difficult, but again the positive aspects of the condition should be emphasized – usually epilepsy is easily controlled, it is not inherited, it does not lead to mental illness, etc. It is also perfectly possible to have a family (see section on pregnancy), and for people with active epilepsy to look after and bring up children. There is a danger of over-dependency in some relationships, and of treating the affected partner as a child; both of these should be avoided.

PSYCHIATRIC DISEASE AND EPILEPSY

The connection between psychiatric disease and seizures is complex. In the past, epilepsy was viewed as a form of psychiatric disease, but now it is considered a physical brain disease. Psychiatric disease is, however, not uncommon in people with epilepsy. A person with epilepsy faces many social pressures, and is more likely to be unemployed and single. It is thus not surprising that anxiety and depression are common in those with epilepsy, especially those with a long history of poorly controlled seizures. However, both seizures and antiepileptic drugs can compound this depression through their effects on the brain, and can occasionally themselves produce a very severe depression that may require hospitalization and drug treatment.

Rarely, patients with temporal lobe epilepsy have episodes of paranoia and schizophrenic-like illnesses. These episodes are usually short lived occurring around the time of a seizure, just after a seizure or between seizures. In a few these episodes may persist, and may require long-term drug treatment. The exact association between temporal lobe epilepsy and psychosis is unclear, because both increases in seizure frequency (flurries of seizures) and decreases in seizure frequency can in some cases result in psychotic episodes.

Some psychiatric diseases and epilepsy have a common cause, for instance severe brain damage at birth may lead to seizures, personality problems and psychiatric disease. In these cases, it is not the epilepsy that causes the psychiatric problems but the underlying cause that results in both.

KEY POINTS

√ All people who have a driving licence need to inform the DVLA if they develop epileptic seizures

√ It is advisable to inform an employer if you have epilepsy

√ High-risk situations such as strenuous or dangerous sports should be avoided; most sports can be enjoyed under some supervision

√ Parents should not over-protect their children with epilepsy because this can result in social isolation

√ Forming relationships can occasionally be difficult for people with epilepsy, but people with epilepsy must be careful not to let the condition 'control' their lives

Overall outlook

CHANCES OF SEIZURES STOPPING

The outlook or prognosis of a condition is the 'forecast' for that condition; it tells us what is going to happen in the future. As was described in the introduction, epilepsy resolves in most people, and can thus be said to have a good prognosis. About 80 per cent of people on antiepileptic medication become seizure free, and there thus has to be the decision about when to stop the medication. It is usual to wait for a patient to be seizure free for roughly two years before stopping medication. There are a number of factors that determine the chances of success or failure in withdrawing drugs, including the underlying cause of the epilepsy. Overall, however, about 60 per cent of patients who have been seizure free for two years successfully come off drugs.

The chances of coming off medication are better in the young, and in those taking only one antiepileptic drug. Some people do not wish to risk coming off their drugs, because the social consequences of having a seizure may be too great (loss of driving licence, etc.).

These social consequences tend to be greater in adults than in children. Indeed, because of the better chances of withdrawing medication, the lesser consequences of having a seizure and the effects of medication on schooling, seizure-free children are often the group that benefit most from coming off their antiepileptic drugs.

One of the questions that has been the subject of debate for many years is whether antiepileptic drugs themselves help cure the condition as well as stopping seizures. The answer to this question is unknown. Recently, however, studies have demonstrated that even late antiepileptic drug treatment probably carries the same good prognosis as early drug treatment.

MENTAL AND PHYSICAL HEALTH

There is often concern that epilepsy and seizures commonly lead to mental and physical deterioration. This is not so. In most cases, seizures either stop or are well controlled by antiepileptic drugs, and these people usually lead normal lives. Unfortunately, there are a few who have uncontrolled seizures, in whom mental and physical deterioration may occasionally be seen. In these cases, however, the deterioration is usually due to the underlying cause of the epilepsy or injuries that occur during the seizures rather than the seizures themselves.

The development of mental illness is often another concern, but, as has already been explained, mental illness directly attributable to seizures is rare, and seizures themselves rarely lead to the destruction of personality and mind.

DEATH AND EPILEPSY

This is a sensitive issue that many patients and doctors ignore. The question, however, often remains in people's minds – does epilepsy affect life expectancy? The answer is that poorly controlled, severe epilepsy most certainly does, and even people with well-controlled epilepsy may have a slightly shortened life expectancy. The reasons for this are not altogether certain, but in a number of cases the underlying cause of the epilepsy (e.g. a brain tumour) may obviously shorten life expectancy.

In addition, people with epilepsy are at a higher risk of accidents usually while having a seizure or as the result of the seizure. There may also be socioeconomic factors at play. Sudden unexpected death, which is a sudden unwitnessed death in a previously healthy person for which no cause is found post mortem, is more common in epilepsy and may be as high as one in 400 people with epilepsy per year (probably even higher in people with severe epilepsy). The reasons for this are again unclear, but it may be the result of an unwitnessed seizure.

Having said this, most seizures are entirely innocent – they do not result in death or brain damage.

What, however, is certain is that people with well-controlled epilepsy do better than those with poorly controlled epilepsy, and as our treatment of epilepsy continues to improve so the prognosis for epilepsy, the lives of those with epilepsy and even the life expectancy of those with epilepsy improve along with it.

KEY POINTS

√ Epilepsy resolves in most people

√ People with epilepsy can control or stop their seizures with drugs and can then lead normal lives

√ Most seizures are entirely innocent, rarely causing brain damage or death

Epilogue

In this book there are a number of important points that we would like to emphasize.

- Epilepsy is a common and treatable condition.
- A seizure results from an 'electrical storm' in the brain and the form of a seizure depends on where it starts and how far it spreads.
- A number of conditions can be confused with seizures.
- There are a multitude of causes of seizures.
- Febrile convulsions rarely lead to epilepsy.
- Most people with epilepsy are well controlled with drug treatment, which must be taken regularly.
- Doses of antiepileptic drugs are determined by the balance of seizure control against drug side effects.
- Antiepileptic blood levels are merely a guide to drug doses.
- Epilepsy gets better and 'goes away' in many people.
- The prognosis probably relates to the underlying cause of the epilepsy.
- Brain surgery is successful in and suitable for a number of patients with drug-resistant epilepsy.
- Most prejudice against people with epilepsy is unjust, but often it is not as great as the person with epilepsy believes.
- Most people with epilepsy should lead normal lives, and should not be over-protected.
- Lastly, epileptic is an adjective that should be confined to the phrase 'epileptic seizure' and not be used to describe and stereotype people.

Useful Addresses

ASSESSMENT CENTRES FOR EPILEPSY

In the UK there are a number of specialist assessment centres for epilepsy. Two have been designated for adults (National Hospital – National Society for Epilepsy and Bootham Park Hospital) and one for children (Park Hospital for Children). There are, however, other specialist epilepsy units, including National Hospital for Neurology and Neurosurgery, David Lewis Centre and King's College Hospital. In addition to these, there are specialist units in many regional neurological centres. These units specialise in the assessment of patients with epilepsy, especially those who are resistant to antiepileptic drug treatment.

Bootham Park Hospital
Bootham
York YO3 7BY
Telephone: 01904 610777

David Lewis Centre
Alderley Edge, Mobberley
Cheshire SK9 7UD
Telephone: 0156 587 2613

King's College Hospital – Epilepsy Unit
Denmark Hill, London SE5 8AZ
Telephone: 0171 703 6333

National Hospital for Neurology and Neurosurgery – Epilepsy Unit
Queen Square, London WC1N 3BG
Telephone: 0171 837 3611

National Hospital – National Society for Epilepsy
Chalfont Centre for Epilepsy
Chalfont St Peter
Buckinghamshire SL9 ORJ
Telephone: 01494 873991

Park Hospital for Children
Old Road, Headington
Oxford OX3 7LQ
Telephone: 01865 741717

SPECIAL SCHOOLS FOR CHILDREN WITH EPILEPSY

Most children with epilepsy receive

mainstream schooling. There are, however, children with severe epilepsy, learning difficulties or behavioural problems that preclude them from mainstream education. These children are often eligible for residential schooling in a specialist centre where there is medical supervision. A list is given below.

David Lewis Centre
Alderley Edge
Mobberley
Cheshire SK9 7UD
Telephone: 0156 587 2613

St Piers School
St Piers Lane
Lingfield
Surrey RH7 6PW
Telephone: 01342 832243

St Elizabeth's School
Much Hadham
Hertfordshire SG10 6EW
Telephone: 0127 984 3451

EPILEPSY ORGANIZATIONS

There are a number of charitable organizations (listed below) that are involved in providing information about epilepsy, educating the general public about epilepsy, organizing meetings and funding research. Some of these organizations are able to provide videos and information packages for schools. They also run information services. The National Society for Epilepsy is the main association in the UK, and has a local community network.

National Society for Epilepsy
Chalfont Centre for Epilepsy
Chalfont St Peter
Buckinghamshire SL9 ORJ
Telephone: 01494 873991

ALSO:

British Epilepsy Association
Anstey House
40 Hanover Square
Leeds LS3 1BE
Telephone: 0113 243 9393
Freephone Helpline: 0800 30 9030

Croydon Epilepsy Society
Stanley Mews
71 Stanley Road
Croydon CRO 3QF
Telephone: 0181 665 1255

Epilepsy Association of Scotland
National Headquarters
48 Govan Road
Glasgow G51 1JL
Telephone: 0141 427 4911

Irish Epilepsy Association
249 Crumlin Road
Dublin 12, Eire
Telephone: 00 353 1455 7500

Mersey Region Epilepsy Association
Glaxo Neurological Centre
Norton Street
Liverpool L3 8LR
Telephone: 0151 298 2666

Wales Epilepsy Association
Ypant Teg
Brynteg
Dolgellau
Gwynedd LL40 1RP
Telephone: 01345 423339

Glossary

Amytal test is the injection of sodium amytal (an anaesthetic) into each half of the brain in turn in order to determine the possible effects of epilepsy surgery on memory and language.

Aura is the warning that may occur before a major seizure or may occur in isolation; it is a simple partial seizure.

Compliance is the act of taking a drug as instructed.

Computed tomography (CT) is a brain scan using X-rays and computer analysis to form pictures of slices through the brain.

Dysplasia is the abnormal development of brain cells.

Electroencephalography (EEG) is the recording of brain waves (the electrical activity within the brain.

Epileptic seizures are also known as fits and are the result of an electrical storm in the brain. They are divided into **partial seizures** (**simple partial**, **complex partial** and **secondary generalized**) which begin in one part of the brain but can spread to other parts, and **generalized seizures** (**tonic–clonic**, **clonic**, **tonic**, **absences** and **myoclonus**) which begin in both halves of the brain at once.

Febrile convulsions are fits that occur in children at the time of fever; they rarely lead to epilepsy.

Hemispheres of the brain are the two halves of the brain, in most of us the left half is 'dominant' and controls language.

Hippocampus is a part of the temporal lobe (see below), which is involved in the formation of memories and which if damaged commonly causes epilepsy.

Hyperventilation is overbreathing which can occasionally be confused with an epileptic seizure.

Idiosyncratic side effects are side effects that occur in only certain people; the most common side effect with antiepileptic drugs is rash.

Lobes of the brain are different parts of the brain determined by position, and each lobe has a particular set of functions; the **frontal lobe** is at the front and deals with movement, the **parietal lobe** is in the middle and deals with sensation, the **occipital lobe** is at the back and deals with sight and the **temporal lobe** is at the side and deals with memory formation.

Magnetic resonance imaging (**MRI**) is the use of a strong magnetic field and radio waves to cause the vibration of atoms that give off energy which is then turned into a very detailed picture of the brain by computer analysis. MRI is much better than CT at detecting brain abnormalities which cause epilepsy.

Monotherapy is the taking of one drug.

Pharmacoresistant epilepsy is also known as **refractory** or **drug-resistant epilepsy** and is epilepsy that is resistant to antiepileptic drug therapy (this applies only to the minority of people with epilepsy).

Photosensitivity is present in about one in twenty people with epilepsy, and is the propensity to have a seizure brought on by flashing lights.

Polytherapy is the taking of two or more drugs.

Prognosis is the 'forecast' for a condition.

Pseudoseizures are seizures that are not epileptic but which are like an emotional outburst usually due to deep-rooted psychological problems. They do not respond to antiepileptic drug treatment, and can be difficult to tell apart from epileptic seizures.

Status epilepticus is a seizure or series of seizures without consciousness being regained that continues for over 30 minutes. If the seizure is a convulsion (convulsive status epilepticus), then this is a medical emergency, and the patient should be taken to hospital.

Syncope is a faint.

Video telemetry is the simultaneous recording of EEG with video, and is used in difficult to diagnose patients and for assessment before epilepsy surgery.

Index